Copyright ©

Table of contents

Introduction

There is a consensus among all clinical specialties that the fat content of the average diet should be lowered to decrease the risk of cardiovascular morbidity and mortality. Low-fat diets are food where 30% or less of the calories come from fat. Multiple correlational studies have related a country's cardiovascular mortality to the food consumption of its population.

A general rule is that if a provides 100 calories and it has 3 grams or less of fat, then it is a low-fat food. Common examples include vegetables, fruits, whole grain cereals, egg whites, chicken and turkey breast without skin, beans, lentils, peas, seafood, and low-fat dairy, among others.

Fats are essential to us, but we need to consume them in a limited amount. The main four types of dietary fats include polyunsaturated, monounsaturated, trans, and saturated fats. These four varieties of fats differ in their physical and chemical structures. The saturated and trans fats are considered solid at room temperature, whereas the mono and polyunsaturated fats are liquid at room temperature. Regardless of their physical and chemical properties, these all different forms of fat provide nine calories for every gram consumed, which is much higher than the amount of energy supplied per gram of carbohydrates or proteins. The saturated and trans fats raise the low-density lipoproteins (LDL) and are considered unhealthy, whereas the monounsaturated fatty acids (MUFA) and polyunsaturated fatty acids (PUFA), which lower LDL, are considered beneficial.

Current National Cholesterol Education Program (NCEP) guidelines for adults based on ATP III (Adult Treatment Panel III) recommends reducing intake of saturated fats to less than 7 % of the total calories and cholesterol to less than 200 mg/day. Guidelines also recommend that polyunsaturated fat constitutes up to 10% of total calories, and monounsaturated fats constitute up to 20% of total calories.

There is abundant literature to suggest that a decrease or modification of serum cholesterol is a possible way to prevent atherosclerosis. Decreasing the amount of fat intake is an effective means of lowering the serum cholesterol concentration. Hence, a low-fat diet has been widely advocated by clinicians for reducing the cardiovascular-related morbidity and mortality of their patients.

Issues of Concern

There have been multiple issues of concern and controversies around the concept of a low-fat diet. The biggest concern with the promotion of the low-fat diet has been that manufacturing companies are touting products labeled as low-fat products, where they are replacing the fat with large amounts of refined carbohydrates, which increase the risk of metabolic disorders and hypertriglyceridemia. Studies are also reporting that diets rich in carbohydrates, and low in unsaturated fat, can also negatively impact lipoprotein risk factors and increase cardiovascular risks.[3] There is also a proposed theory that refined carbohydrates decrease the cardioprotective action of HDL by altering its metabolic functions. There has undoubtedly been a focus on replacing the carbohydrates for fats, but the specificities of the replaced carbohydrates remain poorly defined. These concerns have led to the development of alternative dietary approaches.

Studies have also raised concern over the potential of lowering HDL cholesterol, raising triglycerides, and cause unfavorable postprandial lipemic changes. So much so that the "2013 AHA/ACC Guideline on Lifestyle Management to Reduce Cardiovascular Risk" did not state any recommendations for dietary cholesterol and indicated a lack of sufficient evidence to show that lowering of dietary cholesterol reduces LDL-C (low-density lipoprotein cholesterol) or not.

The 2015 Dietary Guidelines Advisory Committee did not endorse limiting dietary cholesterol to less than 300 mg/dL as presented in their prior editions. The committee made recommendations with a focus on dietary patterns rather than on the macronutrients.

Clinical Significance

Association with Cardiovascular Disease

There has been a direct relationship between dietary fat intake and cardiovascular disease (CVD). Besides, dietary cholesterol has been a focus of considerable attention due to a direct connection between diet and blood cholesterol levels and the subsequent risk for coronary artery disease.

The level of LDL particles is the best predictor of cardiovascular risk. Studies have concluded that saturated fatty acids raised blood cholesterol levels, whereas PUFA's reduced serum cholesterol levels and MUFA's were neutral.

Studies have also found myristic and palmitic acid to have cholesterol elevating effects, whereas stearic acid did not affect the levels. Trans fatty acids are similar to saturated fatty acids in raising cholesterol, as well. The level of saturated fats, trans-fatty acids should be low, and the levels of polyunsaturated fatty acids should be high. The results from the Nurses' Health Study, in which the women who consumed diets low in saturated and trans fatty acids and relatively high in unhydrogenated mono- and polyunsaturated fatty acids had the least risk for cardiovascular outcomes.

Recent studies have reported that in men, the reduction of total fat and saturated fatty acids from 36% and 12% of energy to 27% and 8% of energy, respectively, resulted in a substantial decline in the total and LDL cholesterol levels.. Over the years, although there has been some decline in the percentage of fat intake, there has been a paradoxical increase in the total amount of fat intake, suggesting that the total energy intake has increased. A large part of the U.S. population still consume diets that contain more total and saturated fatty acids than recommended in dietary guidelines, which is an area of concern.

Association with Cancer

The association between dietary fat and the risk of cancer development has had consistent support through multiple studies. There is epidemiologic evidence demonstrating associations between dietary fat intake and breast, prostate, colon, and even lung cancers in humans.

Of those cancers, dietary fat intake has been the most extensively linked with breast cancer. Various mechanisms have been suggested, including conversion of essential fatty acids to short-lived hormone-like lipids, the production of reactive oxygen species that carry the potential to induce changes in the genomic DNA changes, leading to alterations in gene expression.Other potential mechanisms include modifications in the hypothalamus-pituitary axis leading to alterations in hormone levels, the effect on enzyme functions affecting the estrogen, changes in the structure and functioning of the cells, and changes in immune function. Studies have also suggested a positive effect of polyunsaturated fatty acids, especially the omega -3 fatty acids, to have a protective effect against the development of cancers and high animal fat to have the strongest positive correlation for developing these cancers.

One potential mechanism for the relationship between fat intake and prostate cancer include altered levels of sex hormones.Studies have shown that mortality data from colorectal cancer correlated with the consumption of animal fat. Potential mechanisms for a diet and colon cancer link are primarily related to bile acid secretion or intestinal metabolism. Populations that consume foods containing olive oil or oils derived from marine animals and fish have a significantly lower likelihood of developing colon cancer, suggesting again that fat quality is much more important than the type of dietary fat.

Association with Obesity

Obesity is a chronic disease associated with a plethora of comorbidities like diabetes mellitus, dyslipidemia, hypertension, fatty liver, and obstructive sleep apnea, to name a few.It has multiple external and internal influences. Among the many environmental impacts, dietary fat intake is thought to have the strongest association. Energy imbalances result from excessive nutritional intakes along with low levels of physical activity. If we use BMI as the criterion to define obesity, more than one-third of adults in the United States are categorized as overweight or obese. The rate at which obesity is increasing in this country and throughout the world is alarming. The relationship between diet composition and body weight has been studied in various epidemiological studies, including ecologic, cross-sectional, and prospective studies.Most of the cross-sectional studies show that obese patients have a higher intake of energy from fat than people with a healthy BMI. Fat being an energy-dense food contributes to excess calorie ingestion as compared to other foods. There has also been a hypothesis that obese subjects have difficulty oxidizing fat and maybe under oxidizing it compared to their leaner counterparts.Recent data suggest that for a reduction in absolute amounts of fat consumed and a decline in the percentage of total dietary intake at the population level, a concomitant decrease in body weight has not occurred.

Particularly losing weight with this type of diet can help reduce the risk of various health factors such as heart disease, diabetes and strokes. However, there are a number of step to remember to keep it healthy.

Fat has the most calories per gram when compared to carbohydrates and protein, so often reducing fatty foods from your diet will result in a lower calorie intake and therefore, help you lose weight.

However, you shouldn't cut fats completely because they play a vital role within your body. They are necessary to support cell growth, keep your body warm and protect your organs. They also help with the absorption of fat-soluble vitamins like A, D and E.

There are different types of fat you should be aware of. The two main ones are saturated and unsaturated fats.

Unsaturated fats are considered 'good' fats. They are found in foods such as fatty fish, olive oil, avocados, nuts and seeds. These types of fats are healthy for you, helping to cut cholesterol and reduce heart disease.

There are two main types of unsaturated fats are polyunsaturated fats and monosaturated fats. Both are healthy for you, but omega-3 polyunsaturated fatty acids found in oily fish are particularly beneficial.

Saturated fats are considered 'bad' fats. Although the research is mixed on how bad they are, they are generally linked to increases in cholesterol and heart disease. They are commonly found in full-fat dairy and red meat.

Studies find that the total cholesterol and LDL (the "bad") cholesterol decreases when polyunsaturated fat replaces saturated fat.

Although HDL (the good") cholesterol is also reduced, LDL cholesterol is reduced even more. This increases the ratio of good cholesterol to bad cholesterol (3).

Projections indicate coronary heart disease risk reduces by about 10% for each 5% energy substitution

However, these benefits are likely to be underestimated. This is because polyunsaturated fats have other benefits other than reducing cholesterol. These include reduced inflammation and insulin sensitivity improvements

Foods to Eat on a Low Fat Diet Plan

Generally, you'll want to focus on eating whole foods. Although all foods can be part of a healthy diet, it can be a good idea to just focus on eating more on the healthy foods on the list below:

Fruits. E.g apples, pears, oranges. Berries also contain lots of antioxidants

Vegetables. All kinds of vegetables are great, but particularly cruciferous vegetables (e.g broccoli, cauliflower)

Whole grains. E.g brown bread, quinoa, bulgur wheat. These are rich in fiber.

Fatty fish. E.g salmon, mackerel, tuna, herring. These foods contain the most omega-3 fatty acids, an important nutrient in reducing inflammatory diseases.

Beans. E.g haricot, black, red.

Legumes. E.g chickpeas, lentils, peas. Both legumes and beans are great sources of plant-based protein.

Nuts and seeds. E.g almonds, walnuts, pistachios. Flaxseeds and chia seeds are also a great plant-based source of omega-3 fatty acids

Low-fat dairy. E.g milk, eggs, yogurt. Be sure to check the labels for extra added sugar.

Olive oil. Choose extra-virgin varieties, which aren't diluted with cheaper oils.

Lean protein. E.g fish, chicken, turkey. These contain less saturated fats than red meats like beef and pork.

Foods to Limit on a Clean Eating Diet

You shouldn't feel guilty for treating yourself occasionally, but don't make a habit of eating these foods regularly:

Junk foods: fast food and potato chips

Refined carbohydrates: white bread, pasta, crackers, flour tortillas, biscuits

Fried foods: french fries, donuts, fried meats

Sugar-sweetened beverages: soda, tea with added sugar, sports drinks

Processed meats: bacon, canned meat, salami, sausages

Trans fats: vegetable oil and margarine

What's the Best Low Fat Diet?

We recommend following a Mediterranean-style diet if you're looking to follow a low fat diet.

Although it does contain some fat, it is full of the fats you need to eat in order to maintain a balanced and healthy diet. It is also well studied and has an extensive amount of research backing its use.

It encourages the consumption of the foods listed previously such as fruits, vegetables, whole grains, nuts, seeds, legumes, beans, low-fat dairy, fatty fish and other lean protein. Cooking is done predominantly with olive oil instead of butter, which contains lots of saturated fats.

The main characteristics of eating a Mediterranean diet are typical of a balanced diet and include:

High unsaturated-to-saturated fat ratio

High consumption of fruits, vegetables, legumes, nuts and unrefined grains

Increased consumption of fish

Moderate consumption of low-fat dairy (mostly cheese and yogurt)

Limited intake of red meat and processed foods

Many credible organisations suggest following a Mediterranean diet. These include:

Part of the reason it is highly recommended is not just because of the health benefits, but also how easy to is to follow. Finding an eating style you stick to long-term is important so that you don't yoyo between diets and fall back into unhealthy eating habits.

It is ranked so highly because of both how easy it is to follow as well as the scientific research backing its use. This makes it a great choice if you're looking for a healthy diet that you'll actually stick to.

In terms of the specific studies that back the Mediterranean diet, a few studies looking at various health factors have been linked to below:

Lower risk of cardiovascular events, coronary heart disease,

Lower risk of coronary heart disease

Lower risk of developing type 2 diabetes

Lower risk of breast cancer

Lower risk of obesity

Better cognitive function

The Mediterranean diet pyramid below gives a good visual indication of what foods to prioritize.

At the bottom are common staple foods that are to be consumed in large amounts and more frequently. Portion sizes and frequency decline as you go up the pyramid. The pyramid intentionally does not specify recommended weights of foods or calories. It is only meant to provide an overall look at healthy food choices and the relative proportions.

It does this because good health has been attributed to variation within the overall dietary pattern. The more variety you get within the specified relative allowances per category – the better.

Low Fat Diet Meal Plan

Low Fat Diet Sample Menu

In the meal plan are recipes for breakfast, lunch and dinner.

	Breakfast	Lunch	Dinner
Monday	Banana Yogurt Pots	Cannellini Bean Salad	Quick Moussaka
Tuesday	Tomato and Watermelon Salad	Edgy Veggie Wraps	Spicy Tomato Baked Eggs
Wednesday	Blueberry Oats Bowl	Carrot, Orange and Avocado Salad	Salmon with Potatoes and Corn Salad

Thursday Banana Yogurt Pots Mixed Bean Salad   Spiced Carrot and Lentil Soup

Friday Tomato and Watermelon Salad Panzanella Salad Med Chicken, Quinoa and Greek Salad

Saturday Blueberry Oats Bowl Quinoa and Stir Fried Veg Grilled Vegetables with Bean Mash

Sunday Banana Yogurt Pots Moroccan Chickpea Soup Spicy Mediterranean Beet Salad

Snacks are recommended between meal times. Some good snacks include:

A handful of nuts or seeds

A piece of fruit

Carrots or baby carrots

Berries or grapes

Day 1: Monday

Breakfast: Banana Yogurt Pots

Nutrition

Calories – 236

Protein – 14g

Carbs – 32g

Fat – 7g

Prep time: 5 minutes

Ingredients (for 2 people)

225g /⅞ cup Greek yogurt

2 bananas, sliced into chunks

15g / 2 tbsp walnuts, toasted and chopped

Instructions

Place some of the yogurt into the bottom of a glass. Add a layer of banana, then yogurt and repeat. Once the glass is full, scatter with the nuts.

Lunch: Cannellini Bean Salad

Nutrition

Calories – 302

Protein – 20g

Carbs – 54g

Fat – 0g

Prep time: 5 minutes

Ingredients (for 2 people)

600g / 3 cups cannellini beans

70g / ⅜ cup cherry tomatoes, halved

½ red onion, thinly sliced

½ tbsp red wine vinegar

small bunch basil, torn

Instructions

Rinse and drain the beans and mix with the tomatoes, onion and vinegar. Season, then add basil just before serving.

Dinner: Moussaka

Nutrition

Calories – 577

Protein – 27g

Carbs – 46g

Fat – 27g

Prep time + cook time: 30 minutes

Ingredients (for 2 people)

1 tbsp extra virgin olive oil

½ onion, finely chopped

1 garlic clove, finely chopped

250g / 9 oz lean beef mince

200g can / 1 cup chopped tomatoes

1 tbsp tomato purée

1 tsp ground cinnamon

200g can / 1 cup chickpeas

100g pack / ⅔ cup feta cheese, crumbled

Mint (fresh preferable)

Brown bread, to serve

Instructions

Heat the oil in a pan. Add the onion and garlic and fry until soft. Add the mince and fry for 3-4 minutes until browned.

Tip the tomatoes into the pan and stir in the tomato purée and cinnamon, then season. Leave the mince to simmer for 20 minutes. Add the chickpeas halfway through.

 Sprinkle the feta and mint over the mince. Serve with toasted bread.

View 7 Day Low Fat Diet Plan PDF

Day 2: Tuesday

Breakfast: Tomato and Watermelon Salad

Nutrition

Calories – 177

Protein – 5g

Carbs – 13g

Fat – 13g

Prep time + cook time: 5 minutes

Ingredients (for 2 people)

1 tbsp olive oil

1 tbsp red wine vinegar

¼ tsp chilli flakes

1 tbsp chopped mint

120g / ⅝ cup tomatoes, chopped

½ watermelon, cut into chunks

50g / ⅔ cup feta cheese, crumbled

Instructions

For the dressing, Mix the oil, vinegar, chilli flakes and mint and then season.

Put the tomatoes and watermelon into a bowl. Pour over the dressing, add the feta, then serve.

Lunch: Edgy Veggie Wraps

Nutrition

Calories – 310

Protein – 11g

Carbs – 39g

Fat – 11g

Prep time + cook time: 10 minutes

Ingredients (for 2 people)

100g / ½ cup cherry tomatoes

1 cucumber

6 Kalamata olives

2 large wholemeal tortilla wraps

50g / ¼ cup feta cheese

2 tbsp hummus

Instructions

Chop the tomatoes, cut the cucumber into sticks, split the olives and remove the stones.

Heat the tortillas.

Spread the houmous over the wrap. Put the vegetable mix in the middle and roll up.

Dinner: Spicy Tomato Baked Eggs

Nutrition

Calories – 417

Protein – 19g

Carbs – 45g

Fat – 17g

Prep time + cook time: 25 minutes

Ingredients (for 2 people)

1 tbsp olive oil

2 red onions, chopped

1 red chilli, deseeded & chopped

1 garlic clove, sliced

small bunch coriander, stalks and leaves chopped separately

800g can / 4 cups cherry tomatoes

4 eggs

brown bread, to serve

Instructions

Heat the oil in a frying pan with a lid, then cook the onions, chilli, garlic and coriander stalks for 5 minutes until soft. Stir in the tomatoes, then simmer for 8-10 minutes.

Using the back of a large spoon, make 4 dips in the sauce, then crack an egg into each one. Put a lid on the pan, then cook over a low heat for 6-8 mins, until the eggs are done to your liking. Scatter with the coriander leaves and serve with bread.

View 7 Day Low Fat Diet Plan PDF

Day 3: Wednesday

Breakfast: Blueberry Oats Bowl

Nutrition

Calories – 235

Protein – 13g

Carbs – 38g

Fat – 4g

Prep time + cook time: 10 minutes

Ingredients (for 2 people)

60g / ⅔ cup porridge oats

160g / ⅗ cup Greek yogurt

175g / ¾ blueberries

1 tsp honey

Instructions

Put the oats in a pan with 400ml of water. Heat and stir for about 2 minutes. Remove from the heat and add a third of the yogurt.

Tip the blueberries into a pan with the honey and 1 tbsp of water. Gently poach until the blueberries are tender.

Spoon the porridge into bowls and add the remaining yogurt and blueberries.

Lunch: Carrot, Orange and Avocado Salad

Nutrition

Calories – 177

Protein – 5g

Carbs – 13g

Fat – 13g

Prep time + cook time: 5 minutes

Ingredients (for 2 people)

1 orange, plus zest and juice of 1

2 carrots, halved lengthways and sliced with a peeler

35g / 1 ½ cups rocket / arugula

1 avocado, stoned, peeled and sliced

1 tbsp olive oil

Instructions

Cut the segments from 1 of the oranges and put in a bowl with the carrots, rocket/arugula and avocado. Whisk together the orange juice, zest and oil. Toss through the salad, and season.

Dinner: Salmon with Potatoes and Corn Salad

Nutrition

Calories – 479

Protein – 43g

Carbs – 27g

Fat – 21g

Prep time + cook time: 30 minutes

Ingredients (for 2 people)

200g / 1 ⅓ cups baby new potatoes

1 sweetcorn cob

2 skinless salmon fillets

60g / ⅓ cup tomatoes

1 tbsp red wine vinegar

1 tbsp extra-virgin olive oil

Bunch of spring onions/scallions, finely chopped

1 tbsp capers, finely chopped

handful basil leaves

Instructions

Cook potatoes in boiling water until tender, adding corn for

final 5 minutes. Drain & cool.

For the dressing, mix the vinegar, oil, shallot, capers, basil &

seasoning.

Heat grill to high. Rub some dressing on salmon & cook,

skinned side down, for 7-8 minutes. Slice tomatoes & place

on a plate. Slice the potatoes, cut the corn from the cob &

add to plate. Add the salmon & drizzle over the remaining

dressing.

View 7 Day Low Fat Diet Plan PDF

Day 4: Thursday

Breakfast: Banana Yogurt Pots

Lunch: Mixed Bean Salad

Nutrition

Calories – 240

Protein – 11g

Carbs – 22g

Fat – 12g

Prep time + cook time: 10 minutes

Ingredients (for 2 people)

145g / ⅝ cup jar artichoke heart in oil

½ tbsp sundried tomato paste

½ tsp red wine vinegar

200g can / 1 cup cannellini beans, drained and rinsed

150g / ¾ cup tomatoes, quartered

handful Kalamata black olives

2 spring onions, thinly sliced on the diagonal

100g / ⅔ cup feta cheese, crumbled

Instructions

Drain the jar of artichokes, reserving 1-2 tbsp of oil. Add the oil, sun-dried tomato paste and vinegar and stir until smooth. Season to taste.

Chop the artichokes and tip into a bowl. Add the cannellini beans, tomatoes, olives, spring onions and half of the feta cheese. Stir in the artichoke oil mixture and tip into a serving bowl. Crumble over the remaining feta cheese, then serve.

Dinner: Spiced Carrot and Lentil Soup

Nutrition

Calories – 238

Protein – 11g

Carbs – 34g

Fat – 7g

Prep time + cook time: 25 minutes

Ingredients (for 2 people)

1 tsp cumin seeds

pinch chilli flakes

1 tbsp olive oil

300g /2 cups carrots, washed and coarsely grated

70g / ⅓ cup split red lentils

500ml / 2 ¼ cups hot vegetable stock

60ml / ¼ cup milk

Greek yogurt, to serve

Instructions

Heat a large saucepan and dry fry the cumin seeds and chilli flakes for 1 minute. Scoop out about half of the seeds with a spoon and set aside. Add the oil, carrot, lentils, stock and milk to the pan and bring to the boil. Simmer for 15 minutes until the lentils have swollen and softened.

Whizz the soup with a stick blender or in a food processor until smooth. Season to taste and finish with a dollop of Greek yogurt and a sprinkling of the reserved toasted spices.

View 7 Day Low Fat Diet Plan PDF

Day 5: Friday

Breakfast: Tomato and Watermelon Salad

Lunch: Panzanella Salad

Nutrition

Calories – 452

Protein – 6g

Carbs – 37g

Fat – 25g

Prep time + cook time: 10 minutes

Ingredients (for 2 people)

400g / 2 cups tomatoes

1 garlic clove, crushed

1 tbsp capers, drained and rinsed

1 ripe avocado, stoned, peeled and chopped

1 small red onion, very thinly sliced

2 slices of brown bread

2 tbsp olive oil

1 tbsp red wine vinegar

small handful basil leaves

Instructions

Chop the tomatoes and put them in a bowl. Season well and add the garlic, capers, avocado and onion. Mix well and set aside for 10 minutes.

Meanwhile, tear the bread into chunks and place in a bowl. Drizzle over half of the olive oil and half of the vinegar. When ready to serve, scatter tomatoes and basil leaves and drizzle with remaining oil and vinegar. Stir before serving.

Dinner: Med Chicken, Quinoa and Greek Salad

Nutrition

Calories – 473

Protein – 36g

Carbs – 57g

Fat – 25g

Prep time + cook time: 20 minutes

Ingredients (for 2 people)

100g / ⅗ cup quinoa

½ red chilli, deseeded and finely chopped

1 garlic clove, crushed

2 chicken breasts

1 tbsp extra-virgin olive oil

150g / ¾ cup tomatoes, roughly chopped

handful pitted black kalamata olives

½ red onion, finely sliced

50g / ½ cup feta cheese, crumbled

small bunch mint leaves, chopped

juice and zest ½ lemon

Instructions

Cook the quinoa following the pack instructions, then rinse in cold water and drain thoroughly.

Meanwhile, toss the chicken fillets in the olive oil with some seasoning, chilli and garlic. Lay in a hot pan and cook for 3-4 minutes each side or until cooked through. Transfer to a plate and set aside

Next, tip the tomatoes, olives, onion, feta and mint into a bowl. Toss in the cooked quinoa. Stir through the remaining olive oil, lemon juice and zest, and season well. Serve with the chicken on top.

View 7 Day Low Fat Diet Plan PDF

Day 6: Saturday

Breakfast: Blueberry Oats Bowl

Lunch: Quinoa and Stir Fried Veg

Nutrition

Calories – 473

Protein – 11g

Carbs – 56g

Fat – 25g

Prep time + cook time: 30 minutes

Ingredients (for 2 people)

100g / ⅗ cup quinoa

3 tbsp olive oil

1 garlic clove, finely chopped

2 carrots, cut into thin sticks

150g / 1 ⅔ leek, sliced

1 broccoli head, cut into small florets

50g / ¼ cup tomatoes

100ml / ¼ cup vegetable stock

1 tsp tomato purée

juice ½ lemon

Instructions

Cook the quinoa according to pack instructions. Meanwhile, heat 3 tbsp of the oil in a pan, then add the garlic and quickly fry for 1 minute. Throw in the carrots, leeks and broccoli, then stir-fry for 2 minutes until everything is glistening.

Add the tomatoes, mix together the stock and tomato purée, then add to the pan. Cover and cook for 3 minutes. Drain the quinoa and toss in the remaining oil and lemon juice. Divide between warm plates and spoon the vegetables on top.

Dinner: Grilled Vegetables with Bean Mash

Nutrition

Calories – 314

Protein – 19g

Carbs – 33g

Fat – 16g

Prep time + cook time: 40 minutes

Ingredients (for 2 people)

1 pepper, deseeded & quartered

1 aubergine, sliced lengthways

2 courgettes, sliced lengthways

2 tbsp olive oil

For the mash

400g / 2 cups haricot beans, rinsed

1 garlic clove, crushed

100ml / ½ cup vegetable stock

1 tbsp chopped coriander

Instructions

Heat the grill. Arrange the vegetables over a grill pan &brush lightly with oil. Grill until lightly browned, turn them over, brush again with oil, then grill until tender.

Meanwhile, put the beans in a pan with garlic and stock. Bring to the boil, then simmer, uncovered, for 10 minutes. Mash roughly with a potato masher. Divide the vegetables and mash between 2 plates, drizzle over oil and sprinkle with black pepper and coriander.

View 7 Day Low Fat Diet Plan PDF

Day 7: Sunday

Breakfast: Banana Yogurt Pots

Lunch: Moroccan Chickpea Soup

Nutrition

Calories – 408

Protein – 15g

Carbs – 63g

Fat – 11g

Prep time + cook time: 25 minutes

Ingredients (for 2 people)

1 tbsp olive oil

½ medium onion, chopped

1 celery sticks, chopped

1 tsp ground cumin

300ml / 1 ¼ cups hot vegetable stock

200g can / 1 cup chopped tomatoes

200g can / 1 cup chickpeas, rinsed and drained

50g / ¼ cup frozen broad beans

zest and juice ½ lemon

coriander & bread to serve

Instructions

Heat the oil in a saucepan, then fry the onion and celery for 10 minutes until softened. Add the cumin and fry for another minute.

Turn up the heat, then add the stock, tomatoes, chickpeas and black pepper. Simmer for 8 minutes. Add broad beans and lemon juice and cook for a further 2 minutes. Top with lemon zest and coriander.

Dinner: Spicy Mediterranean Beet Salad

Nutrition

Calories – 548

Protein – 23g

Carbs – 58g

Fat – 20g

Prep time + cook time: 40 minutes

Ingredients (for 2 people)

8 raw baby beetroots, or 4 medium, scrubbed

½ tbsp sumac

½ tbsp ground cumin

400g can / 2 cups chickpeas, drained and rinsed

2 tbsp olive oil

½ tsp lemon zest

½ tsp lemon juice

200g / ½ cup Greek yogurt

1 tbsp harissa paste

1 tsp crushed red chilli flakes

mint leaves, chopped, to serve

Instructions

Heat oven to 220C/200C fan/ gas 7. Halve or quarter beetroots depending on size. Mix spices together. On a large baking tray, mix chickpeas and beetroot with the oil. Season with salt & sprinkle over the spices. Mix again. Roast for 30 minutes.

While the vegetables are cooking, mix the lemon zest and juice with the yogurt. Swirl the harissa through and spread into a bowl. Top with the beetroot & chickpeas, and sprinkle with the chilli flakes & mint.

View 7 Day Low Fat Diet Plan PDF

Low Fat Diet Shopping List

This shopping list corresponds to the 7 day plan, serving 2 people. No snacks are included.

View 7 Day Low Fat Diet Plan PDF

Life after the meal plan

Find more recipes on our site

Your journey doesn't end after 7 days of Mediterranean-
style low-fat recipes. It's about finding recipes that can

become staples in your household and creating eating habits that actually last.

We've got plenty of recipes online already. Just use the search function on our home page if you're looking for a specific ingredient or check out our recipe page.

You can also sign up for our 28 day plan for over 100+ recipes and 4 weeks of meal plans.

Disclosure